Self-care For Single Moms

Danny Soap

Published by Eureka Tales, 2023.

SELF-CARE FOR SINGLE MOMS

First edition. September 24, 2023.

ISBN: 979-8223059202

Written by Danny Soap.

Table of Contents

Chapter 1: Introduction

Being a single mom is tough. You've got a lot on your plate, and sometimes it feels like there's no time left for yourself. But here's the thing: taking care of yourself is just as important as taking care of your kids. This book is all about showing you how to do that, step by step.

Let's start by talking about what self-care really means. It's not some fancy, complicated idea. Self-care is all about taking time for yourself, doing things that make you feel good, and keeping yourself healthy, both physically and mentally. It's like giving yourself a little recharge so you can be the best mom you can be.

You might wonder why this is so important. Well, think of it this way: when you're on an airplane, they always tell you to put your own oxygen mask on before helping others. Why? Because if you're not okay, you can't help anyone else. The same goes for being a single mom. If you're not taking care of yourself, it's harder to take care of your kids.

Now, we're not saying you have to go on a spa vacation or spend hours meditating every day. We know you're busy, and life can be crazy. But even with a packed schedule, there are simple things you can do to make sure you don't burn out.

In this book, we're going to break self-care down into easy, manageable steps. We'll talk about how to make self-care a part of your daily life, even when it feels like there's no time. We'll also tackle the guilt that sometimes comes with taking time for yourself. Spoiler alert: you deserve it, and your kids will benefit from it too!

You might have heard some myths about self-care. Some people think it's selfish or that it's only for people with lots of free time and money. We're here to bust those myths. Self-care is for everyone, and it doesn't have to cost a fortune. It can be as simple as taking a few deep breaths, going for a short walk, or enjoying a favorite snack.

This book is your guide to self-care as a single mom. We'll cover a wide range of topics, from managing your time to boosting your emotional well-being. We'll talk about how to build a support system, take care of your physical health, and make self-care a natural part of your life.

We'll also share stories from other single moms who have been through it all. You'll see that you're not alone in your struggles and that self-care can make a real difference.

But remember, this isn't a one-size-fits-all approach. We'll give you ideas and tips, but you get to decide what works best for you. Your self-care journey is unique, just like you and your kids.

So, whether you're a newly single mom or you've been on this journey for a while, this book is for you. It's for every single mom who wants to be the best parent she can be while also taking care of herself.

Are you ready to embark on this self-care journey? We promise it's worth it, and you deserve it. Let's get started!

Chapter 2: The Single Mom's Journey

Being a single mom is not a simple road to travel. It's filled with twists, turns, and challenges that can feel overwhelming at times. But it's also a journey filled with love, strength, and growth. In this chapter, we'll take a closer look at what the single mom's journey really looks like.

Life as a single mom often starts with a big change. It might be a breakup, divorce, or the loss of a partner. Suddenly, you find yourself not just responsible for yourself but also for your children all on your own. It's a lot to take in, and it can be a real shock to the system.

One of the first things you might notice is that there's a lot to do. You're not just a mom; you're also a provider, a problem solver, and a multitasker extraordinaire. You become an expert at juggling schedules, managing finances, and handling household chores. It's like running a marathon every day.

But it's not just the physical tasks that can be challenging. The emotional toll of single parenting can be heavy too. There might be moments when you feel lonely, sad, or even angry. It's okay to feel these emotions; they are a natural part of the journey.

One of the biggest challenges you might face is the feeling of overwhelm. It's like there's never enough time or energy to do everything you need to do. You might worry about how to provide for your kids, how to give them a good life, and how to be there for them emotionally.

Sometimes, it can feel like you're carrying the weight of the world on your shoulders. And in a way, you are. But here's the thing: you're also carrying the love, hopes, and dreams of your children. You're their superhero, even on the tough days.

Despite all the challenges, being a single mom can also be incredibly rewarding. You get to witness your child's first steps, hear their laughter, and share their triumphs. You're the one they look up to, and you're the one who shapes their world.

Through this journey, you'll discover just how strong you are. You'll learn to rely on yourself, trust your instincts, and overcome obstacles you never thought possible. You'll develop resilience that will serve you well, not just as a mom, but in all areas of your life.

It's important to remember that you don't have to go through this journey alone. There's a whole community of single moms out there who have faced similar challenges and triumphed. They understand what you're going through, and they can offer support, advice, and friendship.

As you navigate this journey, self-compassion will become your best friend. There will be days when you doubt yourself or wish you could do more. But remember that you're doing the best you can, and that's more than enough. Be kind to yourself and acknowledge your efforts.

In this book, we're going to explore how self-care fits into your journey as a single mom. We'll show you that taking care of yourself is not selfish; it's a necessity. When you're at your best, you can be the best mom for your children.

So, whether you're just starting this journey or you've been on it for a while, know that you're not alone. Many single moms have walked this path before you and have come out stronger and wiser. Your journey may be challenging, but it's also filled with love, growth, and endless possibilities. You've got this!

Chapter 3: Prioritizing Self-Care

Self-care may sound like a fancy term, but at its core, it's about taking care of yourself. It's about making sure you're in good shape, both physically and mentally. But as a single mom, you might wonder, "Do I really have time for this?" The answer is a resounding yes. In fact, it's not just important; it's necessary. Let's dive into why and how you can prioritize self-care.

Life as a single mom can be hectic, with a never-ending to-do list. From getting the kids ready for school to managing the household, it seems like there's always something demanding your attention. In the midst of all this, your well-being often takes a backseat. But here's the truth: you can't pour from an empty cup.

Imagine you're driving a car on a long road trip. You've got your kids in the backseat, and you're responsible for getting everyone to your destination safely. Now, picture this: you're so focused on driving that you forget to refuel the car. You keep going, thinking you'll fill up the tank later, but eventually, the car sputters to a stop because it's out of gas.

In this analogy, you're the car, and self-care is the fuel. If you neglect self-care, you'll eventually run out of energy, and that's not good for you or your kids. That's why prioritizing self-care isn't a luxury; it's a necessity.

But how do you do it? Here's the secret: you make it a non-negotiable part of your life. Just like you wouldn't skip meals or neglect your kids' needs, you shouldn't skip self-care either. It's not something you do if you have extra time; it's something you make time for, even if it's just a few minutes a day.

Start by recognizing that self-care isn't selfish. It's not taking time away from your kids; it's giving them a healthier, happier mom. When you're well-rested, less stressed, and emotionally balanced, you can be more present for your children. You can listen to their stories, play with them, and offer them the love and support they need.

Self-care isn't just about you; it's a gift you give to your family. So, how can you make it a priority? Here are some steps to get you started:

1. Set Boundaries: It's easy to say yes to every request and obligation that comes your way, but that can leave you feeling overwhelmed. Learn to say no when necessary. Your time is precious, so use it wisely.

2. Schedule Self-Care: Just as you schedule appointments and activities for your kids, schedule self-care time for yourself. It could be a daily walk, a weekly bath, or a monthly treat. Put it on the calendar, and stick to it.

3. Delegate: You don't have to do everything on your own. If your kids are old enough, involve them in household chores. Ask for help from family or friends when needed. Share the load, so you have more time for self-care.

4. Learn to Say No to Guilt: Guilt is a common companion on the self-care journey, but it's not your friend. When you take time for yourself, remind yourself that you're doing it for the well-being of your family. Guilt won't change that fact.

5. Keep It Simple: Self-care doesn't have to be elaborate or expensive. It can be as basic as taking deep breaths, enjoying a cup of tea, or spending a few minutes in quiet reflection. Find what works for you and fits into your daily life.

6. Prioritize Health: Physical health is a crucial aspect of self-care. Make sure you're eating well, staying hydrated, and getting regular exercise. A healthy body supports a healthy mind.

7. Embrace "Me Time": Find moments in your day when you can focus solely on yourself, even if it's just for a few minutes. Use this time to recharge and reset.

8. Seek Support: Reach out to other single moms or support groups. They can offer advice, encouragement, and a sense of camaraderie. Knowing you're not alone in this journey can be incredibly empowering.

9. Reflect and Adjust: Periodically, take a step back to assess how you're doing with your self-care routine. Are you making time for yourself regularly? Are there any adjustments you need to make?

Remember, self-care isn't a one-size-fits-all solution. What works for one person may not work for another, so don't compare yourself to others. Your self-care journey is unique, just like you. The key is to find what brings you joy, relaxation, and rejuvenation.

In the chapters ahead, we'll explore various aspects of self-care in more detail. You'll discover practical tips, strategies, and real-life stories from other single moms who have successfully integrated self-care into their lives. Your journey to prioritizing self-care starts here, and we're here to guide you every step of the way.

Chapter 4: Creating a Self-Care Mindset

Imagine if you had a magic mirror that could show you the most powerful tool for self-care—a positive mindset. In this chapter, we'll explore how your thoughts and attitudes can shape your self-care journey. It's not about turning life into a fairytale, but it is about believing in yourself and making self-care a part of your everyday reality.

1. Embrace the Power of Positivity

Think of positivity as your trusty sidekick on your self-care journey. It's not about ignoring problems or pretending everything is perfect, but it's about focusing on the bright spots in your life. When you approach self-care with a positive mindset, you're more likely to stick with it.

Imagine waking up in the morning and saying to yourself, "Today is a new day, and I can handle whatever comes my way." That simple thought can set the tone for your entire day. Instead of dreading the challenges, you'll be better equipped to face them head-on.

2. Practice Gratitude

Gratitude is like a superpower that can transform your outlook on life. It's all about recognizing and appreciating the good things, no matter how small they may seem. Take a moment each day to think about what you're grateful for. It could be a hug from your child, a sunny day, or a warm meal.

When you focus on the positive aspects of your life, it becomes easier to see the silver linings in challenging situations. Gratitude can shift your perspective and help you find joy even in the midst of difficulties.

3. Be Mindful

Mindfulness is about being present in the moment. It's not about dwelling on the past or worrying about the future. When you practice mindfulness, you tune in to what's happening right now.

As a single mom, life can feel like a whirlwind, with a million things vying for your attention. Mindfulness helps you slow down and savor the present. It's as simple as taking a deep breath and noticing the sights, sounds, and sensations around you.

Mindfulness can be especially helpful during self-care activities. For example, when you take a bath, focus on the feel of the warm water on your skin, the scent of your favorite soap, and the calming sound of the water. It turns a regular bath into a rejuvenating experience.

4. Shift from Guilt to Self-Compassion

Guilt is a sneaky emotion that can creep into your self-care routine. You might feel guilty for taking time for yourself when there are dishes to wash, homework to help with, or bills to pay. But here's the truth: self-care isn't selfish, and you deserve it.

Imagine if a dear friend came to you and said they needed a break. Would you tell them they should feel guilty for taking care of themselves? Of course not! You'd probably encourage them to rest and recharge.

Now, here's the challenge: treat yourself with the same kindness and understanding. When guilt tries to sneak in, remind yourself that self-care is a necessity, not a luxury. You're not neglecting your responsibilities; you're ensuring you have the energy and well-being to meet them.

5. Practice Self-Compassionate Self-Talk

The way you talk to yourself matters more than you might realize. If you're constantly berating yourself for not being a "perfect" mom or for making mistakes, it can take a toll on your self-esteem. Self-compassion involves treating yourself with the same kindness and understanding you'd offer a friend.

Next time you catch yourself being overly critical, try this exercise: pretend you're talking to a friend who's in the same situation. What would you say to her? Now, say those same kind words to yourself. It might feel strange at first, but it's a powerful way to boost your self-esteem and create a self-care mindset.

6. Cultivate a Growth Mindset

A growth mindset is all about believing that you can learn and grow through your experiences, even when they're tough. It's about embracing challenges as opportunities for growth rather than as failures.

As a single mom, you're bound to face challenges. Instead of seeing them as roadblocks, view them as chances to learn and become even more resilient. This mindset shift can make self-care feel like a natural part of your journey.

7. Let Go of Perfectionism

Perfectionism is like a heavy backpack that can weigh you down on your self-care journey. It's the idea that everything must be flawless, and any imperfection is a failure. But here's the truth: perfection is an impossible goal.

Instead of striving for perfection, aim for progress. Understand that it's okay to make mistakes, and it's okay if everything doesn't go according to plan. Self-care isn't about doing everything perfectly; it's about doing your best and taking care of yourself along the way.

8. Surround Yourself with Positivity

The people you surround yourself with can influence your mindset. Seek out friends and support groups that uplift and inspire you. Avoid those who bring negativity or make you doubt your self-worth.

Creating a self-care mindset is like planting a garden. It takes time and effort, but with patience and care, it can bloom beautifully. When you approach self-care with a positive mindset, you'll find it easier to prioritize and integrate into your daily life. Remember, you have the power to shape your thoughts and attitudes, and that power can make your self-care journey not just possible but also enjoyable.

Chapter 5: Time Management and Organization

Time is like a precious coin that we can spend only once, and as a single mom, it often feels like you've got to spend it wisely. Juggling the responsibilities of parenting, work, and self-care can be overwhelming, but with some simple strategies, you can make the most of your time and find moments for self-care.

1. Prioritize Your To-Do List

Imagine your day as a puzzle, and your to-do list as the puzzle pieces. Your job is to fit those pieces together in a way that makes the most sense. Start by identifying the most important tasks that need to be done that day. These are your big puzzle pieces.

Once you have your big pieces in place, you can fill in the gaps with smaller tasks. This approach helps you focus on what truly matters and prevents you from getting overwhelmed by a long list of chores.

2. Create a Daily Schedule

A daily schedule is like a roadmap for your day. It helps you stay on track and ensures you allocate time for self-care. Start by blocking out specific time slots for your most important tasks, like work, childcare, and self-care.

For example, if you work during the day, allocate a block of time in the evening for self-care. It could be as simple as dedicating 30 minutes to read a book, take a bath, or practice a hobby you enjoy. Having a set schedule can help you carve out self-care time, making it a regular part of your routine.

3. Use Time Blocks

Time blocking is a technique where you allocate specific blocks of time for similar tasks. For example, you might set aside a block of time in the morning for work-related tasks, followed by a block for household chores, and then a block for spending time with your children. This method helps you stay focused and efficient.

When it comes to self-care, create a time block dedicated solely to taking care of yourself. Whether it's a short break during the day or a longer period in the evening, having a designated self-care time block ensures you don't forget to prioritize your own well-being.

4. Set Realistic Expectations

It's essential to set realistic expectations for what you can accomplish in a day. As a single mom, you might have a lot on your plate, so it's okay to acknowledge your limitations. Be gentle with yourself and understand that some days, you might not get everything done.

By setting achievable goals and being flexible with your schedule, you reduce stress and create room for self-care. Remember that self-care doesn't have to be time-consuming or elaborate. Even small, intentional moments of self-care can make a significant difference.

5. Delegate and Seek Help

You don't have to do everything on your own. Don't hesitate to delegate tasks to your children if they're old enough to help. It's a valuable way to teach them responsibility and teamwork.

Additionally, reach out to your support network—friends and family who can lend a hand when you need it. Asking for help is a sign of strength, not weakness. It frees up your time and energy for self-care and other important responsibilities.

6. Use Technology Wisely

Technology can be a valuable tool for time management and organization. Consider using apps or digital tools to help you stay organized. You can use calendar apps to schedule appointments, set reminders, and plan your day efficiently.

Moreover, there are apps designed specifically for self-care, offering guided meditation, relaxation exercises, and daily affirmations. These can be handy for incorporating self-care into your routine, even when you have limited time.

7. Create a Weekly Meal Plan

Meal planning can save you a significant amount of time and reduce stress around meal preparation. Take some time each week to plan your family's meals, create a shopping list, and prep ingredients in advance.

When you have a meal plan in place, you won't have to spend precious time every day deciding what to cook or rushing to the grocery store. This frees up time for self-care and ensures that you and your family are eating nutritious meals.

8. Set Up a Family Calendar

A family calendar is a visual tool that can help you keep track of everyone's schedules in one place. You can use it to coordinate appointments, school activities, and work commitments. By having a clear overview of your family's schedule, you can identify pockets of time for self-care.

Include your self-care activities on the family calendar just like any other important appointment. This sends a clear message that self-care is a priority for you and your family.

9. Declutter and Simplify

A cluttered and disorganized environment can make it challenging to manage your time effectively. Take some time to declutter and simplify your living space. Remove items that you no longer need or use, and create a more streamlined and peaceful home.

A clutter-free environment can reduce stress and make it easier to focus on self-care. When your physical space is in order, you'll find it easier to relax and recharge.

10. Practice Time-Blocking for Self-Care

In addition to scheduling self-care, consider implementing time-blocking specifically for self-care activities. Set aside dedicated blocks of time in your calendar for self-care, just as you would for work or appointments.

During these self-care time blocks, focus solely on taking care of yourself. Whether it's a short walk, a mindfulness exercise, or indulging in a favorite hobby, these moments of self-care can be rejuvenating and essential for your well-being.

Remember, time management and organization are tools to help you create space for self-care in your life. By prioritizing your time and responsibilities, you can ensure that self-care becomes a regular and essential part of your routine. It's not about finding more time but using the time you have more efficiently to nurture both yourself and your family.

Chapter 6: Building a Support System

Life as a single mom can sometimes feel like you're navigating uncharted waters. It's a journey filled with ups and downs, challenges, and triumphs. But you don't have to go it alone. Building a support system is like having a team of allies by your side, ready to offer encouragement, advice, and a listening ear. In this chapter, we'll explore the importance of a support system and how to cultivate one.

1. The Power of Connection

Humans are social beings, and we thrive on connection. As a single mom, it's easy to become isolated or feel like you're carrying the weight of the world on your shoulders. But you don't have to bear the load alone. Connecting with others who understand your journey can make a world of difference.

When you have a support system, you have people who can empathize with your experiences, share their own stories, and provide valuable insights. They become your cheerleaders during the tough times and your celebration partners during the good times.

2. Finding Like-Minded Single Moms

One of the most powerful aspects of a support system is the understanding and camaraderie you can find among other single moms. They've walked a similar path, faced similar challenges, and can offer empathy like no one else.

Consider joining local or online support groups for single moms. These communities provide a safe space to share your thoughts, ask for advice, and connect with moms who are on a similar journey. It's a place where you can be heard and understood.

3. Friends and Family

Your friends and family can be a crucial part of your support system. They know you well, and they care about your well-being. Don't hesitate to lean on them when you need assistance or simply a listening ear.

Communicate your needs with your loved ones. Sometimes, they might not know how to help unless you ask. Whether it's watching the kids for a few hours, running errands together, or providing emotional support, your friends and family can play a vital role in your support system.

4. Seek Professional Help When Needed

In addition to friends and family, there are times when professional support is essential. If you're facing challenges related to your mental health, seek the guidance of a therapist or counselor. They can offer tools and strategies to help you cope with stress, anxiety, or any other emotional issues you may be experiencing.

Professional support isn't a sign of weakness; it's a proactive step toward your well-being. Just as you'd see a doctor for a physical ailment, seeing a mental health professional is a way to prioritize your mental and emotional health.

5. Connect with Your Children's School

Your children's school can also be a valuable resource in building your support system. Teachers, counselors, and other school staff members are often willing to provide guidance and support. They can help you navigate any challenges your children may face in their educational journey.

Stay involved in your children's school life by attending parent-teacher conferences, school events, and parent support groups if available.

Building a positive relationship with the school can create a network of support for both you and your children.

6. Online Communities and Resources

The internet has opened up a world of opportunities to connect with others, even if you can't meet in person. There are numerous online communities and resources specifically designed for single moms.

You can join forums, social media groups, or follow blogs and websites dedicated to single parenting. These online spaces provide a platform to seek advice, share experiences, and find encouragement from a global community of single moms.

7. Support for Self-Care

Your support system isn't just there for the tough times; it's also there to help you prioritize self-care. Sometimes, friends or family can step in to provide childcare while you take a break. They can encourage you to schedule self-care time and hold you accountable for taking it.

Self-care is an essential part of your well-being, and having a support system that understands its importance can make it easier to incorporate into your routine. They can even join you in self-care activities, making it a bonding experience for everyone involved.

8. Building Trusting Relationships

As you build your support system, focus on nurturing trust and open communication. Trust is the foundation of any strong relationship, and it's essential in a support system. When you trust the people in your support network, you can be vulnerable and seek help without fear of judgment.

Open communication is equally crucial. Be willing to share your thoughts, feelings, and challenges with your support system. Encourage them to do the same. A two-way flow of communication creates a supportive environment where everyone can benefit.

9. The Reciprocal Nature of Support

Remember that support is a two-way street. Just as you receive support from your network, be prepared to offer support in return. Your experiences and insights can be valuable to others in your support system. Building a reciprocal relationship strengthens the bonds within your network.

Sometimes, offering support to someone else can be as fulfilling as receiving it. It creates a sense of purpose and connection within your support system, fostering a positive and mutually beneficial environment.

10. Recognizing the Value of Your Support System

Your support system isn't just a collection of people; it's a lifeline, a source of strength, and a network of care. It's there to remind you that you're not alone on your journey as a single mom. Embrace the value of your support system, cherish the connections you've built, and continue to nurture those relationships.

In the chapters ahead, we'll delve deeper into specific aspects of self-care and how your support system can play a pivotal role in your self-care journey. Your network of allies is a priceless resource, and together, you can navigate the challenges and celebrate the joys of single motherhood.

Chapter 7: Emotional Well-Being

Emotions are like the colors of the sky, ever-changing and sometimes unpredictable. As a single mom, you may find yourself riding a rollercoaster of feelings. It's okay; your emotions are a natural part of the human experience. In this chapter, we'll explore the importance of emotional well-being and how to navigate the complex landscape of feelings.

1. Acknowledge Your Emotions

Emotions are like messengers, delivering important information about what's happening in your life. They can be like friends telling you how you're doing. Some days, you might feel happiness, love, or contentment, while other days, you might experience sadness, frustration, or even anger.

The first step to emotional well-being is acknowledging your emotions. It's okay to feel whatever you're feeling, without judgment. Emotions aren't good or bad; they just are. By recognizing and accepting your feelings, you gain insight into yourself and your needs.

2. Practice Emotional Awareness

Emotional awareness is the ability to tune in to your feelings, understand where they're coming from, and respond to them appropriately. It's like having a compass that helps you navigate your emotional landscape.

Start by checking in with yourself throughout the day. Ask yourself, "How am I feeling right now?" Give yourself the space to honestly acknowledge your emotions. This practice can help you stay in touch with your inner world and make informed decisions.

3. Embrace Self-Compassion

Self-compassion is like a warm, comforting hug for your soul. It's the practice of treating yourself with kindness and understanding, especially when you're going through tough times. As a single mom, you're bound to face challenges, and self-compassion is your ally in handling them.

Imagine if a dear friend came to you feeling sad or overwhelmed. You'd offer them a listening ear, words of comfort, and a reassuring presence. Now, imagine treating yourself the same way when you're struggling with difficult emotions. Self-compassion is a powerful tool for emotional well-being.

4. Develop Healthy Coping Strategies

Life is full of moments that can trigger a range of emotions. Developing healthy coping strategies is like having a toolkit to navigate these moments effectively. Instead of turning to unhealthy coping mechanisms, like avoidance or numbing, you can choose strategies that support your well-being.

Healthy coping strategies might include talking to a friend or therapist, practicing relaxation techniques, journaling, or engaging in physical activity. These tools can help you manage stress, process difficult emotions, and find balance in your emotional world.

5. Create a Supportive Environment

Your environment plays a significant role in your emotional well-being. Surrounding yourself with a supportive and nurturing atmosphere is like tending to a garden where your emotions can flourish.

Build a network of friends and family who understand and validate your feelings. Share your thoughts and emotions with those you trust, and don't be afraid to seek their support when needed. A supportive environment can provide a safety net during challenging times.

6. Set Boundaries

Setting boundaries is like protecting your emotional space. It's about recognizing your limits and communicating them to others. As a single mom, you may have many responsibilities, but it's essential to prioritize your emotional well-being.

Don't be afraid to say no when you need to. Boundaries are a way of preserving your emotional energy and ensuring that you're not stretched too thin. They empower you to focus on what truly matters to you and your family.

7. Practice Stress Reduction Techniques

Stress is like a storm that can cloud your emotional sky. Finding effective ways to reduce stress is essential for emotional well-being. There are various stress reduction techniques you can explore, such as:

- Deep Breathing: Taking slow, deep breaths can calm your nervous system and reduce stress.

- Meditation and Mindfulness: These practices help you stay present and centered, reducing anxiety and stress.

- Exercise: Physical activity releases endorphins, which are natural mood lifters.

- Creative Outlets: Engaging in creative activities like art, music, or writing can be therapeutic and help release pent-up emotions.

- Nature: Spending time in nature can have a calming and rejuvenating effect on your emotions.

8. Seek Professional Support

There may be times when your emotional well-being requires professional support. Just as you'd see a doctor for a physical ailment, seeking the help of a therapist or counselor is a proactive step toward your emotional health.

A mental health professional can offer guidance, tools, and strategies to help you navigate challenging emotions and life circumstances. Don't hesitate to reach out for help when you need it. It's a courageous and wise choice for your well-being.

9. Practice Gratitude

Gratitude is like a ray of sunshine that can brighten even the cloudiest emotional day. It involves recognizing and appreciating the positive aspects of your life. Cultivating a gratitude practice can shift your focus from what's lacking to what's abundant.

At the end of each day, take a moment to reflect on three things you're grateful for. They can be small or significant, from a warm cup of tea to a heartfelt conversation with your child. Gratitude can bring a sense of joy and balance to your emotional well-being.

10. Embrace Emotional Growth

Emotional well-being isn't about eliminating negative emotions; it's about growing through them. Every emotion you experience is an opportunity for growth and self-discovery. When you face difficult feelings head-on, you become more resilient and emotionally intelligent. As a single mom, you have the strength to navigate the complexities of your emotional world. Embrace your emotional journey, acknowledge your feelings, and remember that your emotions are a valuable part of your human experience.

In the chapters ahead, we'll delve into specific aspects of self-care that support your emotional well-being. You have the capacity to nurture your emotions, cultivate resilience.

Chapter 8: Physical Health and Fitness

Your body is like a trusted companion on your journey as a single mom. It's the vessel that carries you through life's adventures, and taking care of it is essential. In this chapter, we'll explore the importance of physical health and fitness and how you can integrate them into your busy life.

1. The Foundation of Physical Health

Physical health is like the solid ground upon which your life is built. It encompasses various aspects, including nutrition, sleep, hydration, and regular check-ups. Each of these components plays a role in keeping your body strong and resilient.

2. Nourishing Your Body

Imagine your body as a car, and food as the fuel that keeps it running. Choosing nutritious foods is like filling your tank with premium gasoline. It provides your body with the energy, vitamins, and minerals it needs to function optimally.

A balanced diet includes a variety of foods, such as fruits, vegetables, lean proteins, whole grains, and healthy fats. Make an effort to incorporate these into your meals to support your physical health. Remember that small, gradual changes in your diet can lead to long-term benefits.

3. Staying Hydrated

Water is like the elixir of life for your body. It's essential for digestion, circulation, temperature regulation, and overall well-being. Make it a habit to drink enough water throughout the day to stay hydrated.

Carry a reusable water bottle with you to make it convenient to sip water regularly. If you find it challenging to drink plain water, infuse it with slices of fruit or herbs for a refreshing twist.

4. Prioritizing Sleep

Sleep is like a reset button for your body and mind. It's during sleep that your body repairs and rejuvenates itself. As a single mom, it's easy to feel like you're burning the candle at both ends, but prioritizing sleep is essential for your physical health.

Create a bedtime routine that signals to your body that it's time to wind down. This might include activities like reading a book, taking a warm bath, or practicing relaxation techniques. Aim for at least seven to eight hours of quality sleep each night.

5. Regular Check-Ups and Screenings

Just as you wouldn't skip maintenance checks on your car, regular check-ups with healthcare professionals are crucial for your physical health. These visits can help detect and address health issues early, before they become more significant concerns.

Schedule routine appointments with your primary care physician, dentist, and any specialists as needed. Don't forget about screenings like mammograms, pap smears, and vaccinations. Prevention and early detection are key to maintaining your physical health.

6. Physical Activity for Vitality

Physical activity is like the tune-up your body needs to stay in top shape. Regular exercise offers numerous benefits, including increased energy, improved mood, and enhanced overall health. It's also an essential component of maintaining a healthy weight.

Find ways to incorporate physical activity into your daily routine. It doesn't have to be a grueling workout at the gym. Activities like brisk walking, dancing, gardening, or playing with your children all contribute to your physical fitness.

7. Finding Joy in Movement

Exercise doesn't have to feel like a chore; it can be a joyful experience. Think about physical activities you genuinely enjoy and look forward to. When you find joy in movement, it becomes easier to make exercise a regular part of your life.

Whether it's joining a dance class, practicing yoga, or simply going for a bike ride with your kids, find activities that bring you pleasure and make you feel good. The key is to make physical activity a sustainable and enjoyable habit.

8. Setting Realistic Goals

Physical fitness is like a marathon, not a sprint. Setting realistic goals is crucial to long-term success. Avoid the temptation to embark on extreme diets or exercise routines that are unsustainable in the long run. Instead, focus on gradual, achievable changes.

Set specific, measurable goals for your physical health. For example, you might aim to walk for 30 minutes five days a week or incorporate more vegetables into your meals. As you achieve these goals, celebrate your progress and set new ones.

9. Listen to Your Body

Your body is like a wise friend that communicates its needs. Pay attention to the signals it sends you. If you're feeling tired, give yourself permission to rest. If you experience pain or discomfort during exercise, stop and seek guidance from a healthcare professional.

Listening to your body is an essential aspect of physical health. It allows you to make choices that support your well-being and prevent overexertion or injury.

10. Incorporating Physical Health into Your Routine

As a single mom, finding time for physical health can be a challenge. However, it's possible to integrate it into your daily life. Here are some practical tips:

- Family Activities: Involve your children in physical activities. Go for family walks, bike rides, or play active games together.

- Short Bursts: You don't need hours for exercise. Short, intense workouts or even brief, frequent bursts of activity can be effective.

- Multitasking: Combine physical activity with other tasks. For example, you can do squats while cooking or practice deep breathing exercises during a break.

- Schedule It: Treat physical activity as an essential appointment. Block out time in your calendar for exercise, and make it a non-negotiable part of your routine.

- Accountability: Consider partnering with a friend or joining a fitness group. Accountability can motivate you to stay consistent.

Physical health and fitness are like the foundation of a strong, resilient life. When you take care of your body, you have the energy and vitality to face the challenges of single motherhood with confidence. Remember that small, consistent changes can lead to significant improvements in your physical well-being.

Chapter 9: Sleep and Rest

Sleep and rest are like the soothing balm that rejuvenates your body and mind. As a single mom, you may often feel like you're running on empty, but prioritizing quality sleep and rest is essential for your well-being. In this chapter, we'll explore the importance of sleep and rest and how you can make them a non-negotiable part of your life.

1. The Foundation of Well-Being

Imagine sleep as the foundation of a strong and healthy life. It's during sleep that your body repairs and restores itself. Your brain processes information, and your emotions find balance. Quality sleep is like the cornerstone upon which your well-being is built.

2. Understanding Your Sleep Needs

Just as cars have different fuel requirements, individuals have varying sleep needs. Some people thrive on seven hours of sleep, while others may need nine hours to feel their best. Understanding your unique sleep requirements is crucial.

Pay attention to how you feel after different amounts of sleep. Do you wake up feeling refreshed and alert, or do you feel groggy and irritable? Use this awareness to determine your ideal sleep duration.

3. The Importance of a Sleep Schedule

A consistent sleep schedule is like a rhythm that guides your body's internal clock. Going to bed and waking up at the same times each day helps regulate your sleep-wake cycle. This consistency signals to your body when it's time to rest and when it's time to wake up.

As a single mom, it may be challenging to stick to a strict sleep schedule, but do your best to establish a routine. Create a bedtime routine that signals to your body that it's time to wind down. Avoid large variations in your sleep schedule, even on weekends, to maintain a stable sleep pattern.

4. Creating a Restful Sleep Environment

Your sleep environment is like a cozy nest where you can relax and unwind. Make your bedroom a sanctuary for rest. Keep the room cool, dark, and quiet. Invest in a comfortable mattress and pillows that provide adequate support.

Limit exposure to screens, such as phones, tablets, or TVs, before bedtime, as the blue light emitted can interfere with your sleep-wake cycle. Consider using blackout curtains and white noise machines if needed.

5. The Role of Stress and Anxiety

Stress and anxiety are like the thieves that can steal your precious sleep. The demands of single motherhood can often lead to increased stress levels. When you're anxious or worried, it can be challenging to relax and fall asleep.

Practice stress-reduction techniques, such as deep breathing, mindfulness, or meditation, to calm your mind before bedtime. Create a worry journal to jot down your concerns, allowing your mind to release them and prepare for restful sleep.

6. Physical Activity and Sleep

Physical activity is like a lullaby for your body. Regular exercise can improve sleep quality and help you fall asleep faster. However, avoid vigorous exercise too close to bedtime, as it may energize you and disrupt your sleep.

Incorporate physical activity into your daily routine, but aim to finish exercising at least a few hours before bedtime. Activities like walking, yoga, or stretching can be especially beneficial for promoting restful sleep.

7. The Impact of Diet on Sleep

Your diet is like the menu that influences your sleep quality. Be mindful of what you consume, especially in the hours leading up to bedtime. Avoid heavy, spicy, or rich foods that may cause discomfort or indigestion.

Limit caffeine and alcohol intake, especially in the evening. Both substances can interfere with your sleep cycle and reduce sleep quality. Opt for light, soothing snacks if you're hungry before bed, such as a small serving of yogurt or a banana.

8. Evening Wind-Down Routine

An evening wind-down routine is like a gentle lullaby for your body and mind. Engage in calming activities before bedtime to signal to your body that it's time to relax. This routine might include:

- Reading: Enjoy a book or magazine to quiet your mind.

- Warm Bath or Shower: A warm bath can relax your muscles and prepare your body for sleep.

- Soft Music: Listen to soothing music that helps you unwind.

- Mindfulness or Relaxation Exercises: Practice techniques that reduce stress and promote relaxation.

- Herbal Tea: Some herbal teas, like chamomile or lavender, can have a calming effect.

9. Naps and Power Naps

Napping is like a mini-recharge for your body. Short naps, often referred to as power naps, can provide a quick energy boost during the day. Aim for naps that last around 20-30 minutes to avoid feeling groggy.

However, be cautious about long naps, as they can interfere with your nighttime sleep. If you find yourself needing frequent naps, it may be a sign that you're not getting enough quality nighttime sleep.

10. The Connection Between Rest and Productivity

Rest is like the secret weapon that enhances your productivity. When you're well-rested, you're better equipped to handle the challenges of single motherhood. Your mind is sharper, your emotions are more balanced, and your energy levels are higher.

Remember that rest is not a luxury; it's a necessity. Make it a priority in your life, just as you prioritize other responsibilities. Recognize that rest is an investment in your well-being and your ability to be the best mom you can be.

In the chapters ahead, we'll delve into specific self-care practices that support your physical health and promote restful sleep. Sleep and rest are essential pillars of your well-being, and by nurturing them, you're taking a vital step toward a healthier, happier life as a single mom.

Chapter 10: Mental Health and Therapy

Your mental health is like the compass that guides your emotional and psychological well-being. As a single mom, you may encounter various challenges that impact your mental health. In this chapter, we'll explore the importance of mental health and the role of therapy in supporting your emotional well-being.

1. The Significance of Mental Health

Mental health is like the foundation upon which your emotional and psychological well-being is built. It encompasses your thoughts, feelings, and behaviors. Just as you prioritize your physical health, it's essential to pay attention to your mental health.

2. Understanding Your Mental Health

Understanding your mental health is like knowing the landscape of your inner world. It involves recognizing your thoughts, emotions, and reactions. As a single mom, you may experience a wide range of feelings, from joy and fulfillment to stress and frustration.

Take time to reflect on your mental state. Ask yourself how you're feeling, and be honest with your responses. Understanding your mental health is the first step toward nurturing it.

3. The Power of Self-Care

Self-care is like a nurturing embrace for your mental health. It involves practices and activities that support your emotional well-being. As a single mom, self-care is not a luxury; it's a necessity.

Engage in self-care activities that resonate with you. This might include meditation, journaling, spending time in nature, or pursuing hobbies you enjoy. Self-care is a way to recharge and protect your mental health from the demands of daily life.

4. Seeking Professional Support

Professional support is like a guiding light when you're navigating challenging emotional terrain. Therapy or counseling is a valuable resource for addressing mental health concerns. A therapist is like a trusted partner who can help you explore your thoughts and emotions in a safe and confidential space.

Therapy offers various approaches, including cognitive-behavioral therapy (CBT), dialectical behavior therapy (DBT), and talk therapy. Each approach has its focus, but the goal is to help you understand and manage your emotions, improve your coping skills, and enhance your overall mental health.

5. The Benefits of Therapy

Therapy is like a toolbox filled with strategies and techniques to support your mental health. It can provide numerous benefits, such as:

- Emotional Regulation: Therapy can help you identify and manage intense emotions, reducing emotional distress.

- Improved Coping Skills: You'll learn effective ways to cope with stress, anxiety, and other challenges.

- Enhanced Communication: Therapy can improve your communication skills, both in your personal relationships and with your children.

- Conflict Resolution: You'll gain insights into resolving conflicts and navigating difficult situations.

- Increased Self-Awareness: Therapy fosters self-reflection and self-discovery, helping you understand your thought patterns and behaviors.

- Strengthened Relationships: Improved mental health often leads to healthier and more fulfilling relationships with your loved ones.

6. Overcoming Stigma

Stigma is like a shadow that can cast a cloud over seeking help for your mental health. Some individuals may hesitate to explore therapy due to misconceptions or societal stigma surrounding mental health.

Remember that seeking therapy is a courageous and responsible choice. It's a sign of strength to acknowledge when you need support and take steps to prioritize your mental health. Therapy is a tool for growth and well-being, just like any other form of healthcare.

7. Finding the Right Therapist

Finding the right therapist is like discovering a trusted confidant. It's essential to choose a therapist with whom you feel comfortable and understood. Consider the following factors when seeking a therapist:

- Credentials: Ensure that your therapist is licensed and has appropriate credentials.

- Specialization: Look for therapists who specialize in areas that align with your needs, whether it's stress management, parenting challenges, or anxiety.

- Compatibility: Schedule an initial consultation to determine if you feel a connection with the therapist. Trust your instincts when evaluating the therapeutic relationship.

- Approach: Discuss the therapist's approach and methods to ensure they align with your preferences and goals.

- Accessibility: Consider practical factors, such as the therapist's location, availability, and fees.

8. Incorporating Therapy into Your Life

Incorporating therapy into your life is like adding a valuable tool to your self-care toolkit. It's a commitment to your mental health and well-being. Create a schedule that allows you to attend therapy sessions regularly.

Be open and honest during therapy sessions. Your therapist is there to support you and provide guidance. The more you communicate, the more effective the therapeutic process will be.

9. Self-Reflection and Growth

Therapy is like a mirror that reflects your inner world. It's an opportunity for self-reflection and personal growth. Through therapy, you can gain insights into your thought patterns, behaviors, and emotions.

As you work with your therapist, you'll discover new ways to navigate challenges and achieve your goals. Therapy empowers you to make positive changes in your life and enhances your overall well-being.

10. The Journey of Healing

Healing is like a winding path that leads to emotional well-being. Therapy is a significant step on this journey. It's not a destination but a process of self-discovery and growth. Embrace the journey of healing, and remember that you have the strength and resilience to overcome challenges and nurture your mental health.

In the chapters ahead, we'll explore specific self-care practices that complement therapy and support your mental health. By prioritizing your mental well-being and seeking professional support when needed, you're taking a proactive and courageous step toward a healthier and happier life as a single mom.

Chapter 11: Financial Well-Being

Your financial well-being is like the sturdy bridge that supports your journey as a single mom. Managing your finances effectively is essential for providing stability and security for yourself and your children. In this chapter, we'll explore the importance of financial well-being and practical steps to achieve it.

1. The Significance of Financial Well-Being

Financial well-being is like the cornerstone upon which your life is built. It influences various aspects of your daily life, from meeting basic needs like housing and food to planning for your future and your children's education. Taking control of your finances is a vital step toward a brighter future.

2. Assessing Your Financial Situation

Assessing your financial situation is like taking a snapshot of your current financial landscape. Start by gathering information about your income, expenses, debts, and savings. This evaluation will provide you with a clear picture of your financial standing.

List your sources of income, including your job, child support, government assistance, or any other sources. Next, identify your monthly expenses, such as rent or mortgage, utilities, groceries, childcare, and transportation. Don't forget to include occasional expenses like insurance premiums or annual fees.

3. Creating a Budget

Creating a budget is like drawing a roadmap for your financial journey. A budget helps you allocate your income effectively, ensuring that you cover your essential expenses while also saving for the future. Start by categorizing your expenses as follows:

- Fixed Expenses: These are regular, recurring expenses with a consistent amount, like rent or mortgage, utilities, and insurance.

- Variable Expenses: Variable expenses can fluctuate from month to month. They include groceries, transportation, and entertainment.

- Savings and Goals: Allocate a portion of your income to savings and financial goals, such as an emergency fund or retirement.

- Debt Payments: If you have outstanding debts, budget for the required monthly payments.

4. Reducing Unnecessary Expenses

Reducing unnecessary expenses is like trimming the excess weight from your financial plan. Review your budget to identify areas where you can cut back or eliminate expenses. This might involve dining out less frequently, canceling unused subscriptions, or finding more cost-effective alternatives for certain services.

Challenge yourself to differentiate between wants and needs. Focus on covering your essential needs while being mindful of your discretionary spending.

5. Building an Emergency Fund

An emergency fund is like a safety net for unexpected financial challenges. It's essential to set aside money for emergencies, such as medical bills, car repairs, or unexpected home expenses. Aim to build an emergency fund that can cover at least three to six months' worth of living expenses.

Start by allocating a portion of your income to your emergency fund regularly. Treat this fund as a non-negotiable expense, just like any other bill. Over time, your emergency fund will grow, providing you with financial security and peace of mind.

6. Managing Debt Wisely

Debt management is like navigating through a financial maze. If you have outstanding debts, create a plan to manage them effectively. Start by listing your debts, including credit card balances, loans, or any other obligations.

Prioritize paying off high-interest debts first, as they can be particularly costly. Allocate as much of your budget as possible toward debt repayment while making at least the minimum required payments on all your debts. As you pay off one debt, redirect those funds toward the next one, creating a snowball effect.

7. Saving for the Future

Saving for the future is like planting seeds that will grow into a financial garden. Identify your long-term financial goals, such as retirement, your children's education, or homeownership. Allocate a portion of your income toward these goals regularly.

Consider taking advantage of retirement savings accounts, such as a 401(k) or an Individual Retirement Account (IRA), if available. These accounts offer tax advantages and can help you build wealth for your future.

8. Seeking Financial Education

Financial education is like acquiring tools for your financial toolkit. Learning about personal finance, budgeting, investing, and managing debt can empower you to make informed financial decisions. Explore resources, books, online courses, or local workshops that can enhance your financial knowledge.

Don't hesitate to seek advice from financial professionals or counselors if needed. They can provide guidance tailored to your unique financial situation.

9. Exploring Additional Income Streams

Exploring additional income streams is like planting more financial seeds. Look for opportunities to increase your income, such as part-time work, freelance gigs, or pursuing a side business. These additional income sources can provide financial flexibility and help you achieve your goals more quickly.

Be resourceful and consider your skills and interests when exploring income opportunities. Finding a balance between your primary responsibilities and additional income streams is essential to avoid burnout.

10. Tracking Your Progress

Tracking your financial progress is like measuring the distance you've traveled on your journey. Regularly review your budget, savings, and debt repayment to assess how you're doing. Celebrate your milestones, no matter how small, as they represent progress toward your financial well-being.

Adjust your financial plan as needed to accommodate changes in your circumstances or goals. Stay committed to your financial well-being and remember that achieving financial security is a gradual process.

11. Teaching Financial Literacy

Teaching financial literacy to your children is like providing them with a valuable life skill. Educate your children about money, budgeting, saving, and responsible spending. Encourage them to develop healthy financial habits from a young age, setting them on a path toward financial independence and success.

Financial well-being is a fundamental aspect of your life as a single mom. By taking control of your finances, you provide stability and security for yourself and your family. Remember that small, consistent steps toward financial well-being can lead to significant improvements in your financial situation over time.

Chapter 12: Building a Supportive Environment

Creating a supportive environment is like nurturing a garden where your well-being can flourish. As a single mom, you don't have to navigate the challenges of life on your own. In this chapter, we'll explore the importance of building a supportive environment and practical steps to cultivate one.

1. The Power of Your Environment

Your environment is like the canvas upon which your life unfolds. It includes your physical surroundings, your social circle, and the systems and structures that impact your daily life. A supportive environment can be a source of strength and resilience.

2. Nurturing Positive Relationships

Positive relationships are like the pillars that hold up your supportive environment. Surround yourself with friends and family who understand and uplift you. Cultivate relationships that are built on trust, respect, and mutual support.

Share your thoughts, feelings, and challenges with those you trust. Lean on your support system when you need assistance or simply someone to listen. Positive relationships can provide emotional support during difficult times.

3. Setting Boundaries

Setting boundaries is like creating a protective fence around your well-being. Boundaries are essential for maintaining healthy relationships and safeguarding your mental and emotional space. As a single mom, you have limited time and energy, so it's crucial to allocate them wisely.

Communicate your boundaries clearly and respectfully to others. Let them know what you can and cannot commit to. Boundaries empower you to prioritize self-care and your family's needs.

4. Seeking Help When Needed

Seeking help when needed is like reaching out for a lifeline in times of struggle. Don't hesitate to ask for assistance when you're facing challenges that feel overwhelming. It's a sign of strength, not weakness, to seek support.

Whether it's asking a friend for help with childcare, reaching out to a therapist for emotional support, or seeking financial guidance, remember that there are resources available to assist you. Accepting help is a proactive step toward building a supportive environment.

5. Creating a Safe and Nurturing Home

Your home is like the heart of your supportive environment. Make it a safe and nurturing space for yourself and your children. Ensure that it's a place where you can relax, recharge, and find comfort.

Maintain a clean and organized home to reduce stress and create a sense of order. Incorporate elements that bring you joy, such as favorite colors, soothing scents, or sentimental decorations. Your home should be a reflection of your values and a source of comfort.

6. Finding Community and Resources

Community and resources are like the branches that extend your support network. Explore local and online communities for single moms. These groups can provide valuable information, shared experiences, and a sense of belonging.

Research available resources and programs that can assist you in various aspects of single motherhood, from childcare assistance to financial aid. Knowing where to turn for help is an integral part of building a supportive environment.

7. Fostering a Positive Mindset

A positive mindset is like the sunshine that brightens your environment. Cultivate a mindset of optimism and resilience. Focus on solutions rather than dwelling on problems. When faced with challenges, remind yourself of your strengths and past successes.

Practice gratitude by regularly acknowledging the positive aspects of your life. This simple habit can shift your perspective and enhance your overall well-being.

8. Modeling Healthy Behavior

Modeling healthy behavior is like planting seeds of well-being for your children. Your actions and attitudes serve as a powerful example for your kids. Show them how to prioritize self-care, set boundaries, seek help when needed, and cultivate positive relationships.

By modeling healthy behavior, you empower your children to navigate life's challenges with resilience and confidence. You provide them with valuable life skills that will serve them well in the future.

9. Time Management and Organization

Effective time management and organization are like the gears that keep your environment running smoothly. Develop routines and systems that help you manage your responsibilities efficiently. Create schedules and to-do lists to stay organized and on track.

Prioritize tasks based on their importance and deadlines. Allocate time for self-care and quality time with your children. Effective time management can reduce stress and create a more supportive environment.

10. Letting Go of Negativity

Letting go of negativity is like clearing away the clutter in your environment. Negative thoughts, grudges, and judgments can weigh you down and create a toxic atmosphere. Practice forgiveness, both for others and yourself.

Release negative emotions and thoughts through journaling, meditation, or talking to a therapist. When you let go of negativity, you create space for positivity and growth in your environment.

11. Advocating for Yourself

Advocating for yourself is like raising your voice to protect your well-being. Be your own advocate when it comes to your needs and rights. Speak up when you require accommodations or support, whether at work, in your community, or within your family.

Advocating for yourself is a powerful way to ensure that your environment is conducive to your well-being and that of your children. It reinforces the message that your needs are valid and worthy of attention.

12. Celebrating Achievements

Celebrating achievements is like savoring the fruits of your efforts. Take time to acknowledge and celebrate your accomplishments, no matter how small they may seem. Recognize your resilience and progress on your single motherhood journey.

Share your achievements with your support network, and encourage your children to celebrate their successes as well. Celebration is a way to infuse positivity and motivation into your environment.

Building a supportive environment is an ongoing process that can enhance your well-being and strengthen your ability to thrive as a single mom. By nurturing positive relationships, setting boundaries, seeking help when needed, and fostering a positive mindset, you create a nurturing and empowering atmosphere for yourself and your children.

Chapter 13: Self-Care Activities

Self-care activities are like the essential tools in your toolkit for well-being. As a single mom, taking care of yourself is not a luxury; it's a necessity. In this chapter, we'll explore a variety of self-care activities that you can integrate into your daily life to nurture your physical, emotional, and mental health.

1. Mindful Breathing

2. Guided Meditation

3. Yoga

4. Journaling

5. Creative Expression

6. Nature Walks

7. Reading for Pleasure

8. Aromatherapy

9. Warm Baths or Showers

10. Art and Craft Projects

11. Gardening

12. Dancing

13. Connecting with Loved Ones

14. Mindful Eating

15. Music Appreciation

16. Alone Time

17. Exercise

18. Spa Day at Home

19. Positive Affirmations

20. Volunteer Work

21. Healthy Cooking

22. Goal Setting

23. Decluttering

24. Laughter Yoga

25. Mindful Eating

26. Disconnecting from Technology

27. Napping

28. Boundary Setting

29. Self-Compassion Practice

30. Gratitude Journal

31. Visualization

32. Relaxation Techniques

33. Self-Reflective Writing

34. Deep Breathing Exercises

35. Digital Detox

136. Setting Digital Detox Days

137. Celebrating Your Achievements

138. Practicing Kindness Towards Yourself

139. Reflecting on Your Journey

140. Creating a Self-Care Plan

141. Setting Personal Goals for Happiness

142. Embracing Your Inner Strength

143. Practicing Self-Compassion

144. Finding Serenity in Nature

145. Setting Time for Relaxation

146. Reconnecting with Your Dreams

147. Setting Boundaries with Negative Thoughts

148. Treating Yourself with Respect

149. Practicing Gratitude Daily

150. Setting a Self-Care Intention

Choose self-care activities that resonate with you and fit into your schedule. Remember that self-care is an ongoing practice, and it's essential to prioritize it to maintain your well-being as a single mom.

Chapter 14: Balancing Work and Parenting

Balancing work and parenting is like juggling two important aspects of your life. As a single mom, it can be challenging to find harmony between your career responsibilities and your role as a parent. In this chapter, we'll explore practical strategies to help you navigate this delicate balance.

1. Prioritizing Your Child's Needs

2. Creating a Flexible Work Schedule

3. Seeking Support from Your Employer

4. Utilizing Childcare Services

5. Time Management Techniques

6. Establishing Boundaries

7. Focusing on Quality Time

8. Streamlining Household Tasks

9. Nurturing Self-Care

10. Embracing Imperfection

11. Setting Realistic Expectations

12. Communicating with Your Child

13. Emphasizing Positivity

14. Involving Your Child in Decision-Making

15. Practicing Patience

96. Balancing Academic and Social Demands

97. Encouraging Volunteerism

98. Promoting Healthy Sleep Habits

99. Celebrating Achievements

100. Embracing Uniqueness

Balancing work and parenting is a continuous journey that requires patience, adaptability, and dedication. By prioritizing your child's needs, managing your time effectively, seeking support when needed, and nurturing your own well-being, you can find the equilibrium that allows you to thrive both as a dedicated parent and a successful professional.

Chapter 15: Celebrating Your Strength

Your strength is like the unwavering foundation upon which your life as a single mom is built. It's essential to acknowledge and celebrate the resilience, determination, and courage that you possess. In this chapter, we'll explore the significance of celebrating your strength and ways to do so.

1. Embracing Resilience

2. Recognizing Your Accomplishments

3. Praising Your Determination

4. Honoring Your Courage

5. Acknowledging Your Progress

6. Reflecting on Your Journey

7. Finding Joy in Small Wins

8. Fostering Self-Appreciation

9. Nurturing Self-Compassion

10. Embracing Self-Love

11. Practicing Gratitude

12. Affirming Your Worthiness

13. Celebrating Your Unique Qualities

14. Cultivating Inner Strength

15. Sharing Your Story

96. Reinforcing Your Inner Sanctuary

97. Recognizing Your Inner Brilliance

98. Nurturing Your Inner Sanctuary

99. Setting Your Inner Compass

100. Embracing Your Unique Path

Celebrating your strength is an ongoing practice that can empower you to thrive as a single mom. By acknowledging your resilience, embracing self-compassion, nurturing self-love, and reflecting on your journey, you can find inspiration and motivation to face life's challenges with confidence and grace. Remember that your strength is a source of pride and a testament to your remarkable journey.

Dedication: To Single Mothers, the Unwavering Heroes of Life

This final chapter is dedicated to you, the incredible single mothers who exemplify strength, resilience, and unwavering determination. You are the unsung heroes of life, and your journey is a testament to the remarkable power of the human spirit.

In the face of adversity, you have stood tall, a beacon of hope and inspiration. You've navigated the challenges of single motherhood with grace and courage, proving time and again that love knows no bounds.

You've worn many hats - a provider, a nurturer, a protector, and a mentor. Your role is multifaceted, and your dedication to your children knows no limits. You've sacrificed sleep, personal time, and sometimes even dreams, all to ensure that your children have the best possible chance at a bright future.

Your resilience is awe-inspiring. You've weathered storms, both literal and metaphorical, and emerged stronger each time. Life may have thrown you curveballs, but you've faced them head-on, with determination etched into every step you take.

Your love is boundless. It's the kind of love that lifts you up in the darkest of moments and fuels your spirit with a fierce protectiveness. You've loved, nurtured, and supported your children, often with little recognition or thanks, but always with an unwavering commitment.

Your journey is a testament to the incredible strength that resides within you. You've shattered stereotypes, defied expectations, and rewritten the narrative of what it means to be a mother. Your life is a story of triumph over adversity, a living testament to the incredible power of the human heart.

You've shown the world that being a single mother is not a limitation but a superpower. Your ability to balance work, parenting, self-care, and dreams is a marvel. You've taught your children the value of hard work, resilience, and the importance of never giving up.

Your sacrifices have not gone unnoticed. Your dedication has not gone unappreciated. Your love has not gone unfelt. You are a source of inspiration to your children, your community, and to the world.

In the moments when self-doubt creeps in, remember this: you are stronger than you realize, more resilient than you can imagine, and your love knows no bounds. Your journey is a beacon of hope, a testament to the power of love, and a reminder that, in the face of adversity, you can and will overcome.

To every single mother working tirelessly to provide, nurture, and love, this book is dedicated to you. Your strength, your love, and your unwavering dedication are acknowledged and celebrated. You are not alone on this journey, and your resilience is a source of inspiration for all.

Keep moving forward, keep believing in yourself, and keep celebrating your incredible strength. You are a hero, a warrior, and an embodiment of love. Your journey is a testament to the extraordinary heights that a single mother's heart can reach.

With deepest admiration and respect,

Danny Soap

Also by Danny Soap

Self-care For Single Moms

Watch for more at https://www.buymeacoffee.com/eurekatales.

About the Author

"Self-Care for Single Moms" is a heartfelt and practical guide that celebrates the remarkable strength of single mothers while providing essential insights and strategies for their well-being. Through 15 engaging chapters, it delves into the significance of self-care, creating a supportive environment, effective time management, and nurturing emotional and physical health. With a focus on simplicity and empowerment, this book offers a lifeline to single mothers, reminding them that self-care is not selfish but a vital act of love for both themselves and their children. It serves as a beacon of hope and encouragement, helping single moms navigate the challenges of life with resilience and grace.

Read more at https://www.buymeacoffee.com/eurekatales.